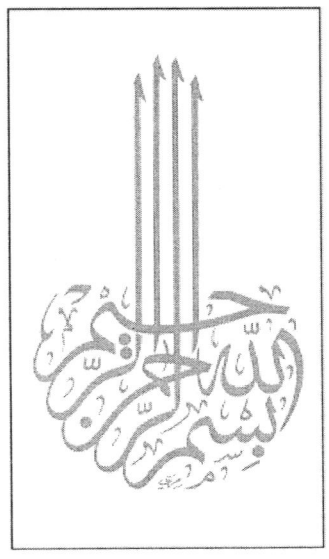

My Personal Experience with Breast Cancer

Nabila Allam

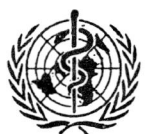

World Health Organization
Regional Office for the Eastern Mediterranean
Cairo 2003

WHO Library Cataloguing in Publication Data

Allam, Nabila

My personal experience with breast cancer / by Nabila Allam.
p.
ISBN 92-9021-318-3
1. Breast Neoplasms   2. Personal Narratives   I.Title
II. WHO Regional Office for the Eastern Mediterranean
[NLM Classification: WP 870]

First published 1986

The World Health Organization welcomes requests for permission to reproduce or translate its publications, in part or in full. Applications and enquiries should be addressed to the Director, General Management, World Health Organization, Regional Office for the Eastern Mediterranean, PO Box 7608, Nasr City, Cairo 11371, Egypt, who will be glad to provide the latest information on any changes made to the text, plans for new editions, and reprints and translations already available.

© **World Health Organization, 2003**

Publications of the World Health Organization enjoy copyright protection in accordance with the provisions of Protocol 2 of the Universal Copyright Convention. All rights reserved.

The designations employed and the presentation of the material in this publication do not imply the expression of any opinion whatsoever on the part of the Secretariat of the World Health Organization concerning the legal status of any country, territory, city or area or of its authorities, or concerning the delimitations of its frontiers or boundaries.

The mention of specific companies or of certain manufacturers' products does not imply that they are endorsed or recommended by the World Health Organization in preference to others of a similar nature that are not mentioned.

The author alone is responsible for the views expressed in this publication.

Cover design and layout by Hazem Sakr
Printed by Concord Press

"...an informed patient gets better faster, frequently is less anxious and is better able to monitor his condition, reports unusual side effects and cooperates with the medical team..."*

---

* *"Ethics and Modern Medicine", Encyclopedia Year Book 1984*

For Hazem & Omar
My sons
Aly & Kamel
My grand-sons

Contents

Special Thanks 8
Acknowledgements 9
Special Acknowledgements 10
Author's Note 11
The Incident 13
"Something … Naughty" 17
Mastectomy 21
My Face 23
Back on my Feet 25
Sweet Home 27
The "Spill-Over" 28
Geneva … Again 30
The Decision 33
Fragile "Please Handle with Care"! 35
My Question Answered 38
Medical Clearance 44
Geneva … Again and Again 46
Nostalgia 49
The Healthier Side of Life 51

Special Thanks

Special thanks to Dar Akhbar El Yom, for taking the initiative and the care of publishing at their expense the 1986 Arabic edition of the book.

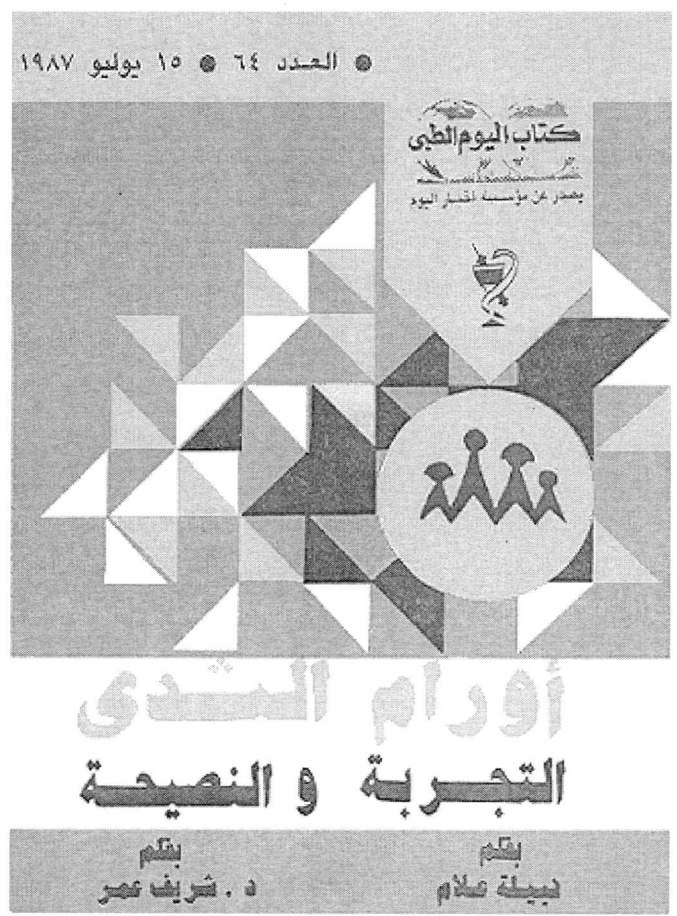

Acknowledgements

When I thought that I had lost contact with words and pencils, Dr M.H. Khayat, who from the very start has believed in this work, encouraged me to review the 1986 edition of my book so as to bring it forth to the year 2003, for WHO to publish it as a useful tool.

Taken to the task, what was believed to have been lost came to light once more. My memory bloomed, the flow of words was extensive and my pencil became my friend again. I am happy to have put forward this work and look ahead for its appearance. I thank Dr Khayat for letting me undergo a more satisfactory use of my time.

Credit goes to Dr Najeeb Al-Shorbaji who made my day, when he put me on the right track to meet the right persons and made the right suggestions.

I will always remember Dr Omer Suleiman for having given me the idea to write my experience, pressing and urging me to do it! But the trouble with good ideas is that they always generate hard work.

I was lucky to be befriended by Professor Sherif Omar who has greatly enriched this book by his generous contribution.

Special thanks go to Jane Nicholson for taking good care of my English once more; Nagwa Allam for the Arabic translation of the 1986 edition; and to Ahmed Hassanein for his constructive advice.

Grateful recognition goes to the Head of Lloyd's Register, Alexandria, for opening wide the doors of the premises, allowing me the facilities to proceed with the booklet; and to "Aya" for her patience, devotion and efficiency in bringing the work to its final new look.

I am also indebted to all those who have participated in organizing my humble work.

Special Acknowledgements

Most touching was the letter received from the American Cancer Society in New York, commenting on the 1986 edition of my book.

"Dear Mrs Allam... Thank you so much for so kindly sharing with us your lovely, sensitive book 'My Personal Experience with Breast Cancer....' I read it with great interest, understanding and admiration. Your courage and optimism came through as shining beacons! A 'Joie de vivre' like yours makes life especially meaningful and wonderful. You are an example to all of us.

While reading it, however, I wondered to myself why you had not been put into contact with specialists in Egypt -- at the Cancer Institute in Cairo as well as in Alexandria. You can imagine how pleased I was when, reading on, I learned of your meeting with Dr Sherif Omar, who is well known to the American Cancer Society. Egypt is indeed well equipped to fight the disease, and has many skilled cancer specialists.

I hope your booklet will be distributed widely in your country. It will greatly help Egyptian women (and their men) not only to understand breast cancer, but also to realize that all cancers are diseases that should be discussed and understood -- and most importantly, that they are treatable if diagnosed in early stages.

It would be wonderful if you could be involved in a rehabilitation program for the benefit of Egyptian women who have been - or will be - treated for breast cancer.

I was also greatly impressed by the sentence in your booklet: "Studying my face will not emphasize the absolute urgency of the need for a cancer awareness programme in Egypt. " How can we help establish such a program? ..."

signed *Gerry S. de Harven, Vice President for International Activities".*

Author's Note

The suggestion of writing about my experience with breast cancer, frankly, shocked me at first! Then, gradually, it aroused in me two contradictory feelings. One part of me completely refused the idea. The other, was gently talking me into accepting it!

On the one hand I immediately perceived the demands that would be imposed upon me and my family, if, such an experience was to be revealed. Not only would I have to open the door and let others see into that part of my private life, but I would also have to bring to light the reactions and attitudes of the people who were involved with me at that turning point in my life. Moreover, I would have no choice except to disclose my personal inner feelings. None of this was easy for me to do.

On the other hand the merits of revealing such an experience were very clear. It might help to ease a fear; it would help to point out that breast cancer today has many choices and is very different from the breast cancer of yesterday. It is curable, if detected early, it may be controlled, lived with, and, even met with a smile! As time passed by, I became heart and soul in favor for this argument.

However, I do not want to seduce you into believing that cancer is just another form of influenza, for example! No, I am only trying to offer my personal experience with the hope that it might succeed in bringing a smile to the faces of those who need it, as well as hope to those, who, one day, might have to face the reality of breast cancer.

The Incident

"Things that do not kill you, might actually strengthen you"

Anon

Nabila Allam is my name, Egypt is my country and, optimistic is my nature. I am in my late forties although people say I look thirty I am married to a wonderful man and the mother of two lovely boys aged twenty-two and sixteen. Delivery of my babies was easy and normal. I had always been healthy and was always what you might call a sports girl; I held the title of ladies squash champion in 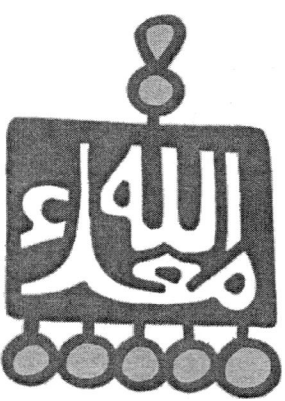 Alexandria for several years during the seventies, also from the age of twelve I swam, played tennis and hockey. Before joining The World Health Organization in June 1983, I worked for seventeen years with Lloyd's Register of London, as the administrative assistant of their Alexandria office. And, in 1979, at age 40 as per the Egyptian Social Insurance System, I qualified for early retirement. I preferred it that way, and was already leading a relaxed and quiet life.

* * *

Where shall I start my story or rather the story of my experience with that illness? The illness which one thinks only happens to others, never to you. I think I will start with that sunny day in March 1982 when I was preparing myself to enjoy a cup of coffee at the Alexandria Sporting Club.

Hand painting offered by artist Mouna Bassili

While dressing my hand happened to touch a little almond shaped lump, so hard, that I could not miss it. Amazingly, I suspected it at once, and in a fraction of a second my brain functioned faster than any sophisticated computer. Everything I had ever read in magazines came back to me quite clearly: the lump in the breast ... the importance of seeing a surgeon immediately ... the drastic results if not faced or reported ... and the hope for survival if detected and treated at an early stage.

All this flooded into my mind but still, I chased such unpleasant thoughts and said to myself, "No ... no ... it can't be that..."

I put on my clothes and set off in my car, but, curiously, instead of heading at Sporting Club, I found myself heading downtown for a surgeon! Waiting at the clinic the drum beats of my heart could be heard at Sporting Club, or maybe a bit further.

"Madam," my surgeon said, "You are an educated woman... you will probably understand..." I understood at once, no escape this was "it". "You are at a critical age" continued the doctor, "I must operate tomorrow or at the latest the day after, to find out whether it is a malignant, or a benign tumor..." "And if it is malignant?" I asked. "Mastectomy, will be the only solution," replied my doctor.

I am sure that what would most interest you now is how I took it. Well, strange but true, once the reality was revealed, I felt no fear, no panic, only a feeling of calmness overwhelmed me at that moment, the reason for which I cannot explain, it is far beyond my knowledge and understanding. Although, here in my country people call it the "illness of death". They never pronounce the name, they say "it". Even I, never mention the name, but refer to it as "it"; you cannot blame me, that's my upbringing and part of my education, but you will see how I was eventually taught to pronounce the word "cancer". I have never had what you might call cancer awareness. In my country, people refuse to talk about it or even discuss it. They are convinced that it is the "no hope" illness; if you have "it" then death, and death alone, is the cure.

* * *

Back home, my husband lent me a shoulder to cry on. Then the two of us fell into a dreadful silence. Upon regaining his norm he said,
- The doctor was hard on you!
- No, not at all ... I prefer it that way and respect him for it ... what matters now is the operation ... here or abroad? ... can we afford it or not?
- "You'll be treated abroad" said my husband, "no matter what the expense, just give me time to settle things."

Time? What time was he talking about? For me, the countdown had begun and cancer was my challenger in that game. I knew the marathon had started, and the winner would be the faster.

"No", I said, "No time must be lost. From this very minute, I will move, I will take over all the arrangements for our departure".

So it happened.

* * *

I immediately phoned a good friend of ours in Geneva and asked him to fix an appointment in two days time with any surgeon he saw appropriate.

Out of curiosity and wishful thinking too, I then visited another surgeon that same afternoon, whose diagnosis, thank God, I preferred not to believe. He pricked the lump with a syringe, no fluid came out. His diagnosis was "no malignancy - no need for surgical intervention". His exact words were "99.5% this is a benign case." I should add here, that my mother out of her love to me, preferred the no-malignancy diagnosis and tried to convince me not to go abroad and to believe the optimistic doctor, or if need be, be operated on in Egypt. Her last attempt to cling onto me was her unforgettable words "... But people in Switzerland die too ... don't they", "Oh, Mom!". I screamed, "Don't discourage me". Yet, I was amazed at her impulsive desire to keep me close to her. May God bless her soul.

That same afternoon, I also consulted a neighbour, a well-known cardiologist who bluntly rejected the 99.5% diagnosis and determined that in such a case fractions of risks cannot be left to chance, but matters should be squared up either in black or in white. His advice was, "If you can afford the expense and can manage to travel within a week, that would be the best solution, but if travel arrangements will make things drag and linger, then treatment in Egypt would be best".

We did manage to get things to run smoothly and quickly. That same night my husband travelled to his farm to settle his affairs whilst I myself travelled to Cairo to obtain our entry visas for Switzerland. Next afternoon the suitcases were ready for the unexpected voyage.

At that point, I felt a pressing need to talk to God. I went to the reception room of our home – why the reception room, I don't know. I closed the sliding doors and conversed with Him for almost an hour and, finally I asked Him to help me accept what cannot be changed. I opened the door. A new strength was born in me. Now I could face life and death. But I can never tell whether this tower of strength that was newly built in me was a direct result of fear or whether it was the credo of hope.

"Something ... Naughty"

"Chances rule men and not men chances"
Herodotus

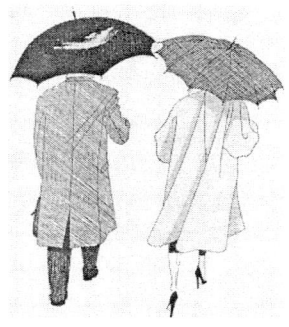

Received at the airport of beautiful Geneva, we learnt that the appointment was fixed in two hours time. Meanwhile, our host took us for lunch "Chez Roberto" – one of those nice Italian restaurants. To my surprise, he had also invited two other couples. "My God," I said to myself "Doesn't he realize that one doesn't like to see anybody at such moments". Nevertheless, it was well thought of, for at times, during lunch, the idea of having cancer, of undergoing lengthy and tiresome treatment would mingle with the creamy lasagna and the chocolate sauce of the ice cream, but then it would quickly bubble away with their interesting conversation.

Then, the moment came to meet the Swiss surgeon. He examined the lump, enquired about the bruise which now covered the lump and which must have occurred after I had seen the second surgeon in Alexandria. "He shouldn't have inserted a needle into the lump", commented the doctor, "the lump is obviously hard".

I feel I should add here that I too made an examination of my doctor and my saviour! Yes, to be honest, at that time, I saw him as both a doctor and a saviour. He had a relaxed smiling face, and gave one the feeling that one could talk, and say anything one might wish to say ... he would have the time for it ... he did not rush ... he did not seem to be saying, "Come on, come out with it, I have other patients waiting". He was careful with each word he pronounced.

I imagine, he was thinking of what would be the best way to deal with this "oriental" woman, perhaps someone had briefed him that in the East people use flowery gentle words, especially tailored to suit such circumstances. Just as I had been told that the European doctors, "especially German and Swiss ones" they said, "wear iron-masked faces, use clumsy words and do not care about one's feelings".

How wrong they were. With the Swiss doctors and nurses I saw only affection and care; I saw medicine practised in the most competent way; I saw the commandments of all religions practised. "Be merciful", they were. "Help your fellow-men", they did. "Don't be hard and clumsy", they never were. "Be clean", the cleanliness of the Swiss hospitals is indeed a fairy tale. And the words of our Prophet, "Be gentle with women, they are fragile", to call them only gentle would belittle their qualities.

– "Doctor," I said. "What's your diagnosis?"
– "I cannot give a final judgment now", replied the doctor, "but, I may say that superficial examination shows 70% malignancy".
– "And the solution?" I asked.
– Well, with your consent you will undergo surgery, I will remove the lump and the pathologist next door will analyse it on the spot whilst you are still under anaesthesia."

Here, he stopped, and was again careful in the choice of his words. He looked straight in my eyes,
– "Then, if we find something ... something naughty for example".
– "NAUGHTY"! I said, "You mean malignant"?

He seemed then relieved and continued,

Well, if we may call things by their proper names, that would be better for everyone". He went on, "If biopsy proves negative, only the lump will be removed, if positive, the whole breast should be removed. The sample will be further examined in the laboratories to determine the condition of the lymph nodes ... if also positive for malignancy, you will also receive other types of treatment ... it could be chemotherapy or radiation therapy or may be both, this will be decided upon by the specialists, if the need arises".

I listened carefully to his words, like a schoolgirl, not allowing one single word to escape, for his words simply meant my being or not being, my quality of life, my whole existence. All I knew about such treatment were the vague notions picked up at social gatherings and in newspapers. Chemotherapy, for example, they connected with loss of hair; radiotherapy, besides loss of hair, they involved with burns, weakness, vomiting and sometimes severe depression.

I now know, from my own personal experience with radiotherapy, that cancer awareness among educated women in Egypt leaves much to be desired. Improvement in our awareness of the disease has only come during the last couple of years

My doctor had also something important to add. He explained that nowadays, one has the choice between mastectomy and radiation therapy, depending of course on the type of cancer, its location and size ... That's why the treating doctor should be trusted to judge what is best for his patient ... because it seems that some women refuse mastectomy under any circumstances, others – when the case allows – prefer radiation, whilst the majority, choose complete removal of the breast.

– So, Madam, you can tell me now what you wish? or in a few hours time if you want to think about it.
– What am I supposed to say? I inquired.
– You tell me, if it is a case of malignancy, do a mastectomy, if there is a choice, do either. You could also say ... do what you think best for me.

Do, what you think best for me, was my spontaneous answer.

I was hospitalized that same afternoon

* * *

Before I proceed any further, I must speak of the attitude of my husband at this turning point in my life. Starting from the moment we left Cairo Airport, he was very calm; he had never interfered in any decision I had taken. He was convinced that this was a critical and decisive moment in my life and that the choice should be left to the party concerned. He behaved very normally, as if nothing had happened, he listened to his music, he read his newspapers, he never lost his "special" sense of humour ... and when given the choice and permission to share my room in hospital, we agreed that it would be better for him to go back to the hotel.

He kissed me goodnight, and left me to my favourite magazines which he had brought me with his newspapers. His relaxed and, at the same time, loving behaviour, consolidated the calmness that had overwhelmed me since the beginning and which still dominates me.

Mastectomy

"God heals, and the Doctor takes the Fees"

Benjamin Franklin

10.30 next morning,

I was wheeled in for the operation. I recall now that the last words I heard before entering the operating theatre were the words of our good friend in Geneva. "Nabila" he said, "all I can tell you at this moment, is that you are in the best of hands". Indeed I was.

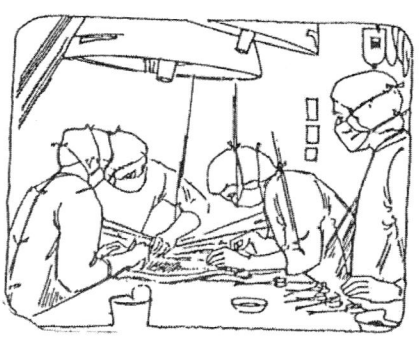

The big clock in the intensive care room clearly showed 3.30 p.m. when, still drowsy, I opened my eyes. "Five hours must have passed away" I thought. My quick calculation and assessment of my case was spontaneous and sharp.

"So, it is cancer ... and they must have removed the whole breast" I imagined. "Yes, it was a malignant tumour, but in its very early stage" said my husband when I had fully recovered from the anaesthesia. "In your case, the doctor preferred mastectomy, and in two days time, we will know the condition of the lymph nodes, then ..." But, my silent running tears stopped him from proceeding further. My thoughts and feelings had slowly left him, quitting his sphere and entering into my own imaginary world.

At that moment, I imagined that I had only a few months to live ... I would not see my eldest son's graduation day ... I would not watch the younger one growing up ... they would grow up on their own ... they would recall our dear old days ... and might sometimes say "We wish mother was here". At that moment I also thought – don't laugh now – I thought that if I die my husband will remarry, and already, I hated him for it! That night I cried my heart out, but it was only for one night, and no more after that night.

A strong beat in my heart woke me up suddenly in the middle of the night. I felt the room was turning upside-down and a strong hand was pulling me down into a deep cavity whilst another, opposing power was resisting that force and eventually succeeded in bringing me back to normal. Everything happened so quickly that I will never be able to feel whether it was a dream or a reality. But I can say that the "touch" of that moment never left me. It is always vivid and clear in my mind.

I rang the bell for the nurse ... I was sweating and exhausted, as if I had been jogging or playing a hard game of squash. I told the nurse what had happened. She was gentle and comforting. And, opening the window to let more fresh air in the room she said, "most probably you have been dreaming". However, being conscientious, she did not fail to report this seemingly minor incident to my doctor, and he gave it special attention and investigations.

My Face

"... and it sorts of helps your case and, it sorts of rests your face ... just smiling"

from EMROSA

6.00 o'clock next morning

    A cheerful young nurse woke me up.

- Come on young lady, up with me to the bathroom, I'll help you with your bath, then we'll make up this nice face.
- What? a bath? Already. No, I don't want it.
- "But why not?" she inquired.
- First of all, I'll catch cold, second I don't feel like it.
- "First" she said "the room and the bathroom are heated so you'll never catch cold; second, taking a bath is like brushing one's teeth, we have to do it whether we feel like it or not; third" she added, "looking nice, and I am sure you'll agree with me, is the pleasure of any woman".

    So, this friendly nurse helped me with my bath and kept me company while I made my face up, a face which only the night before, had been the shelter of so many tears. A face that from now on everyone would want to decipher. I know my people, they would much prefer reading that open-book, my face, rather than talking to me about what's hidden in their own minds. They would never understand that my face is a difficult book for them to read, and that the simplest way would be to talk to it, rather than to try and read it. In trying to read my face, they would never grasp that I am well briefed. To me, cancer is neither taboo nor secret. It is an illness like any other, it has its mortality rate as well as its rate of cure. Looking only at my face, will let go their chance of knowing that the likelihood of curing cancer is greatest when it is diagnosed at an early stage, while it is still localized. Reading my face, will not help them perceive that the sentence "*while it is still localized*" is the key and the critical difference, if the treatment of cancer is to be successful. Studying my face will not emphasize the absolute urgency of the need for a cancer awareness programme in Egypt. Very true, faces we see, hearts we know not.

    Back in my room at hospital the attempts of the friendly nurse to make things look lively and normal in less than twenty four hours after the operation must have succeeded, for, looking in the mirror, my FACE was not bad! And when my husband popped in, even his calm could not in any way, hide his surprise at seeing me already looking so well and already having flowers and listening to soft music!

Back on my Feet

"All that we see and seem, is but a dream within a dream"

Edgar Allen Poe

Two days later we celebrated the safe condition of the lymph nodes, and, four days after I was already sitting on a wooden bench admiring the beauty and quietness of Lac Léman. I even went window-shopping with my husband, furthermore, I tried-out a nice blue dress. It was then that I caught my husband staring at me! I asked him whether he liked the dress, he said "No ... I like your courage."

Then, my thoughts wandered in many directions. The past, the present and the future. As for the past, I could not forgive myself for having had such little knowledge of the most feared disease, the disease which one in ten women will have to deal with at some point of her lifetime. I had never known what a woman should do to detect breast cancer at its earliest and most curable stage. I was never told that a regular six-month check-up by a physician is a must, and that the simplest means of detecting breast cancer is by monthly self-examination, as a physician once put it 'breast topography would make women well-acquainted with their breasts and help them discover any unusual lumps'. As for the present, I longed to be back home, nothing more. Whilst for the future I outlined sketches in my imagination, I would make the most of my life whether it was to be short or long. I would not be afraid of death. I die everyday in my sleep and it is not frightening. I would not make a drama of my life, and that was the most important issue.

In ten days time, I was back on my feet, recovering and ready to resume normal life. Before my departure the doctor briefed me well. He stressed the fact that if there was any suspicion in the other breast, I should not have a mammography, but that if I wished, I could be sent to a centre of excellence in the United States of America for examination. At that time they possessed, in his opinion, the most suitable, up-to-date machine for that type of detection. He added proudly that Switzerland would have this machine in three years time. He asked me to keep him informed of any unusual symptom, however minor it might seem to be and, recommended, that for a one-year period, I be examined monthly by both a physician and a surgeon.

On asking him why I had lost the sense of feeling under my arm, he informed me that it is because he had eradicated the nodes in that particular area for prophylactic purposes. He also advised me not to try lifting heavy objects with that arm to avoid unnecessary worry about possible resulting pain.

He added that such incidents should be put behind one and that one should look well ahead. He also told me that he admired my courage.

At this stage, I can guess the question you might have in mind. The intimate question. The woman-to-woman question.

Well, no. Not at all. I am a woman.

Sweet Home

"Happiness is no laughing matter"

R. Whately

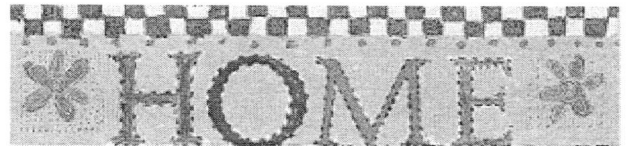

    Landing in Cairo Airport, there they all were, waiting for "the body". Yes, my family was in mourning, waiting for my dead body. They had already condemned me to death and their efforts to hide their sorrow and tears failed them. "Cry" I told them. "Feel free, don't frustrate yourselves", and it was a show! a unique one, a body watching the tears and sorrow of its mourners. They were really confused, my family. They did not know whether they should cry, laugh or smile.

    Back in Alexandria, the behaviour of my children was completely different. They did not come to the airport, which was better, but at home they received me with smiling faces, flowers, chocolates, and the words 'talk to us about it whenever you feel like it'. So natural, and so beautiful.

* * *

    After my return, one question always preoccupied my mind. What would be the approach and results of a breast cancer case treated locally in Egypt? I was completely unaware that the recent rapid progress in this field had already resulted in the adoption of new approaches and techniques in the early detection and diagnosis of breast cancer. The answer to my question was not to come until a few years later!

The "Spill-Over"

"A great part of courage is the courage of having done the thing before"

R. Emerson

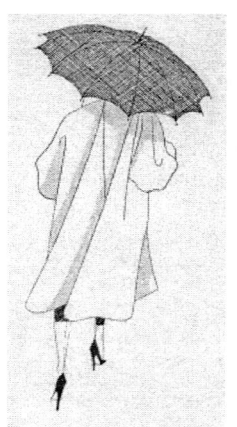

For eight months everyday life continued smoothly and undisturbed. Until one night, sleeping on my side, I felt it again, a lump! I touched it at once, it was hard and at the very end of the incision. I put on the light. It was past midnight. I woke my husband, who said "In the morning we'll see the doctor". I didn't listen, I did not care what time it was, with my nightgown on, I ran up the stairs to our neighbour, the cardiologist. He examined the lump, then called on his wife, the radiologist, they exchanged looks, and calmly he said, "Nabila, I'm not a surgeon"! At once I understood, it was "it" again.

The following morning my surgeon confirmed the suspicion but said that he was not worried and that this is what they call a "spill-over" from the operation, for sometimes, a few cells escape during surgery which is why one school of thought favours automatic radiation therapy after mastectomy to save the trouble and worry of such an incident, whilst another school prefers to deal with it, when and if it occurs, because radiation affects both normal and malignant tissues. "What am I going to go through now Doctor?" I enquired. The surgeon recommended that the lump be removed under local anaesthesia and, as a prophylactic measure, the whole area should be exposed to radiation.

I telexed the diagnosis and recommendations to my doctor in Switzerland. Two hours later I received the following answer "Very optimistic, come tomorrow"!!

* * *

Here, I wish my readers to know that this time I made my trip to Geneva alone. I faced what had to be faced alone. I would take any big and decisive decisions alone.

My husband could not travel at such short notice, he needed four days to square up things, as he put it at the time, but when I re-telexed my doctor "May I come in four days time?" His answer was only two words: "preferably tomorrow". Although "tomorrow" was Christmas, still, his sense of duty came first. For him, tomorrow meant tomorrow.

Geneva ... Again

"Wherever the storm carries me, I go a willing guest"

Horace

The following day Geneva received me beautifully, it was whiter than white, brighter than bright, it took my breath and mind away. It was Geneva on Christmas day. Nevertheless, what should be must be. I was hospitalized and operated on under local anaesthesia. They covered my body and masked my face. Nevertheless, the sense of reckoning and assessing could neither be concealed nor covered up.

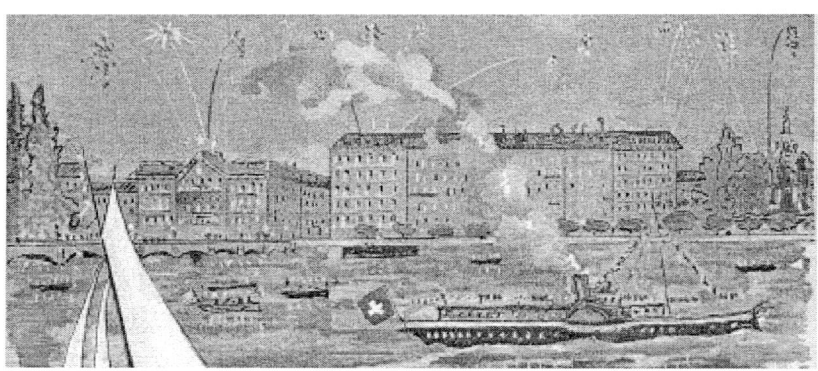

At times, I could feel some "hammering" and "digging" into the very right end of my chest near my right arm. Other times, I would hear the surgeon asking for a specific tool. Yet, what supersedes any imagination is when I heard him ask for a "taxi"! I am not talking nonsense, yes, he did. He said it with a firm and clear tone, "Taxi". "Damn it" I thought, he wants to put himself in a taxi and run home while I am still on the operating table. But immediately and quickly, because of one's need to maintain a human image of the healer, and for the necessity of not being disappointed in one's treating doctor, I gave him allowance, in anticipating that today is Christmas day and that he may be already late for the family lunch. All these notions occurred to me while I was still on the operating table!

The plain point of fact was that the "taxi" had been ordered while I was still in the operating theatre in order to take the sample removed from the new small lump to be analysed on the spot, in a specific laboratory, happening to be open on Christmas day!

The next day, in my room in hospital, and while having a special Christmas lunch prepared by the hospital for all its patients, the surgeon entered my room, my heart bumped. I looked him in the eyes and enquired about yesterday's biopsy "C'est la même chose" replied the doctor and continuing, "in spite of anything, I wish you a merry Christmas and a happy new year, and enjoy your lunch".

Before my departure my doctor reassured me that my condition was under control, but for the prophylactic measures, he recommended that in three weeks time, an eight-week course of radiotherapy treatment which might be combined with chemotherapy – depending on the recommendations of the specialists in both fields – must be applied. He said he would refer me to one of the leading professors in this field who would recommend the relevant programme to be applied here or at home, whichever was the more convenient to me.

Here, I recalled the image most people have of these therapies ... loss of hair, burns, weakness, etc., etc., and, at the end death in pain. I did not conceal my thoughts, I spoke out. "Doctor", I said, "I pity myself for all the miseries I will have to endure." He quickly took the floor. "You must be talking of one or two years back, since then new technologies have been introduced in these fields, and a highly qualified therapist is now able to select the best type of radiation for the situation. The latest radiation equipment has a monitor to ensure that radiation is limited to the cells of the tumour and there are computers, which are now used to determine the doses necessary for treatment. Malaise and other side-effects are, in general, complications of the past." I thanked him and informed him that I would telex him my decision in a week from home.

The Decision

"Fate holds the strings, and men like children move..."

G. Granville

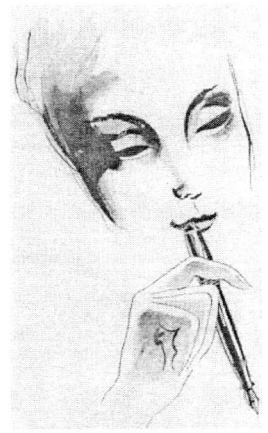

In my hotel room, alone, the decision was already made before I flew back home. I realized at that moment that what I wanted most was to give myself every chance. The whole situation had suddenly become critical. I asked myself, "Where do you think your best chance lies?" "Treatment in Geneva" was the immediate answer. Here I stopped and thought of the many factors that this decision would entail: returning in three weeks time, living in Switzerland for three months; undergoing a lengthy treatment with God only knowing what side-effects it could bring; interrupting my life and that of my family, not to mention the worry they would sustain during my long absence and, the extensive cost we would have to go through. I stopped at this last fact: the cost. Having no health insurance, I made a quick estimation. "My God," I thought, "I'll need quite a handsome fortune of Swiss Francs. What if my husband cannot afford it?" I thought hard and mobilized all the grey cells that I possess, and finally took the decision that I would not let my chance for life escape.

I would go back home, sell my diamond wedding ring, realize my savings account and dispense with the new car which I had bought only few months ago. These together could offer me the type and standard of treatment I wished to have.

Samuel Butler was right, I thought, when he said, "It costs a lot of money to die comfortably." Well, I like to live comfortably and would also like to die in the same style!"

Once home, I informed my husband of my decision. He smiled and said "I may afford the money but not the time". I fully understood his position; one needs the time to make the money. I expressed my gratitude to him and at the same time my regret for the small fortune he would have to spare. His comforting answer came like a soothing remedy, "I am not spending my money," he said "I am investing it in a better Nabila!"

We could have saved a fortune had I known, at that time, the capabilities of Egypt in this sensitive field; I knew nothing of the new trends and modern ideas which were already being implemented and which were advancing along with the latest knowledge of breast cancer. What was missing then, and is still missing, is the publicizing of the information in question.

Fragile "Please Handle with Care"!
"Each man is a hero and an oracle to somebody"
Emerson

Three weeks passed quickly and I returned to my second city, beautiful Geneva. Before starting my treatment I met the radiotherapy Professor. They say he is one of the best in the world in his field. My file was now in front of him. I was struck by the way he was holding the file and how he was turning the pages. Believe me, he treated it like a sacred book, so you can imagine, how I myself was treated! At times, he made me feel as if I was made of fine and rare crystal which he did not want any one to break. At other times, I imagined he wanted to protect me with the label "fragile ... please handle with care"! "If your liver and bones prove cancer-free... I will cure you." He seemed confident. I must say, his words brought into me a new life and a new hope.

For one week, and before the treatment started, I went through all types of investigations and examinations, visited luxurious "palaces of disease", was shunted from one sophisticated machine to another. My blood was tested, my bones and my liver were delivered to giant apparatus, my height was measured, my weight was checked, my teeth and my eyes were not forgotten. Different people of different cultures and different faces intruded on my body. Every bit of my poor little self was pricked and scanned. Finally, the big machines finished their job and sentenced me "not guilty", that is to say, my liver and my bones were cancer free.

The professor talked to me about my liver "Madam ... it is rare to find a liver in such a good condition. This is indeed one of the best results I have run across during my career apropos a liver examination". Amazed, I inquired the reason, "Maybe because it is *alcohol-free*" stressed the master.

A daily five-minute radiotherapy was applied for two continuous months. I also went through what is called a "linear accelerator". The radiology technicians were not only skilled in using the 'giant equipment' and in delivering the prescribed dose of radiation, but one feels that they had also been trained to deal with that most sophisticated machine, the "human" one. One day, one of the radiology team asked me about my favourite singer. Next morning she had brought me the book "Julio by Julio"! In fact I have all the songs Julio Iglesias has ever sung.

I was not burnt, I did not lose one hair, I never felt like committing suicide, I had a good appetite and with the help of the Swiss chocolates and the incredible dairy products, I returned home with seven extra kilograms, some of which, unfortunately, I have not yet managed to lose, although my doctor insists I must. However, the physician recommended that in my case, an average of 10% "fats" above normal standards should always be preserved.

No chemotherapy was recommended in my case.

I spent three months in Geneva, receiving the best of treatment, love and care. I made the most of my stay. The astrologers say that Geminis celebrate events, whatever the events may be. Well, I am a Gemini, and so I made my stay in Geneva a holiday rather than a melancholy. While there, my friends and family overwhelmed me with their telephone calls from Egypt. My husband stayed with me for the first two weeks, and then came back at the end to accompany me back home. My sister and my sister-in-law, each came in turn for a two-week visit. I learnt later that my husband offered them the plane tickets. We used to go sightseeing and, occasionally would go out of town to eat in "gourmet" restaurants.

Believe me, I enjoyed my medical treatment and became skilled in the art of doing nothing.

I returned to my family three months later, safe and sound. My condition was corrected again.

I decided to work. I became a staff member of the World Health Organization, at the Regional Office for the Eastern Mediterranean, at that time based in Aelxandria. At first it was on a temporary basis, as in accordance with the decision of the Joint Medical Service of the United Nations System, in my case I must have a good healthy five-year period, after mastectomy, before a 'Laissez-Passer', no, I mean, a "Medical Clearance" could be granted. I was happy there; I liked my job and my colleagues. I participated in all their social activities. And I joined a few colleagues to practise yoga. We were taught how to relax our bodies, minds and souls. I edited "EMROSA", the WHO/EMR Staff Association's Newsletter which received high praise by both the staff and the officials of the Organization.

I did a lot of globetrotting. Among other places, I have visited the United States of America, Canada, and all of Europe as well as Russia, Japan, China, Korea and India. And lately God granted me the permission to visit his Holy Lands and honoured me with the "Hajj". Very close and within His shrines, I asked for four particular wishes. The four of them have been granted.

I never forgot to have my regular medical check-ups. Every three months I visited both my surgeon and physician in Alexandria, and once a year I went for a complete medical check-up in Geneva. I never failed to report an abnormal symptom.

My Question Answered

"It is a wise father that knows his own child"

Shakespeare

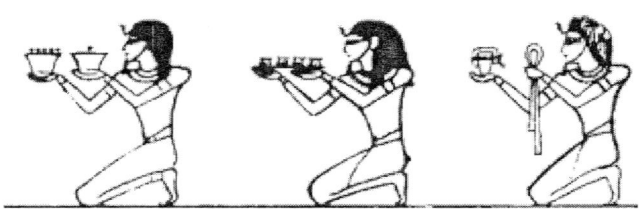

In spite of having received the best possible treatment I could have wished for, and in spite of having resumed a healthy and normal life, still the question of what my country, Egypt had to offer for a case of breast cancer turned over continually in my mind. I truly cared to know the answer.

Four years later, I found the answer! It came by sheer coincidence during the coffee-break of the 'Regional Advisory Panel on Cancer' which was held at the WHO premises in Alexandria. There, I recognized a face whose picture I had frequently seen in local newspapers and on television round-table programmes. I was face to face with Dr Sherif Omar, Professor of Surgical Oncology at the Cancer Institute of Cairo University. Moreover, I remembered having read that his interest nowadays is in research on breast cancer. The 'QUESTION' suddenly flashed back into my mind. I would not let this opportunity escape. I introduced myself to him immediately and, over a cup of coffee, I learnt more and more about the malady and was made aware of how well equipped Egypt is to fight the disease.

I realized at once that Dr Omar's main concern was to stress the importance of a woman to acquire the good habit of examining her breasts in the mirror each month at the end of her menses, so that she may discover any changes in the skin, lumps, discharge from the nipples or change in their contour. For these, he said, can be the manifestations of cancer, but may also be innocent lesions. I understood why it was so vital to report immediately any suspected abnormality to a doctor for advice.

Luckily enough for the Egyptian girl, it might come to pass that the curriculum of the secondary education for girls will include the teaching of breast self-examination.

The Egyptian doctor talked of the good news relating to breast cancer in Egypt; highlighted the modifications which have now been adopted in the techniques of surgery; focused upon the progress attained in diagnosis as well as upon the results of therapy in locally treated cases. And, was optimistic about what is known as 'hormonal knowledge', a new approach which may help control the advance of the cancer. As for 'Chemotherapy', he emphasized the advancement reached in the production of pharmaceuticals that have now much lessened the side effects, including the no-longer loss of hair. Only then did I learn that Egypt now possessed new radiotherapy equipment and modern cobalt machines that greatly enhance the chances of cure, and the hope for cure.

"Recurrence" which is something almost inevitable in the course of the disease, and which causes great concern to the cancer patient, is also well looked after locally. If discovered early enough, and followed-up efficiently by a physician, the condition of the patient could be corrected again.

The general appearance of the Egyptian woman who has had a mastectomy was not overlooked by the Egyptian team. Plastic surgery would provide them with a new breast, in moulded plastic, while the other breast could be operated on to make it look exactly like the new one. Thus the appearance of the patient will be normal, and even better than normal, "... we will eventually give her the breast of her early twenties." added the Professor wittily!

Not through with all the good news, Dr Sherif Omar was keen and enthusiastic in stating his opinion that, cancer should be considered like any ordinary disease; its hazards and risks, being less than, for example, those of kidney, liver or heart disease. He would like us to think of cancer as a common disease in our community, like mild diabetes, for example, which can be lived with, and controlled. And with the large amounts of money pouring into cancer research and the extensive research being carried out as a result, we may even achieve better results than with any other disease in the world.

Not only that, but he is also calling upon the linguists to find for us another word for "cancer"... the word is disliked because of its past history and does not represent the nature of the disease any more.

Don't you think, it was really worthwhile waiting four years for such an answer?!

Breast self-examination
From a pamphlet produced by the Memorial Sloan-Kettering Cancer Center

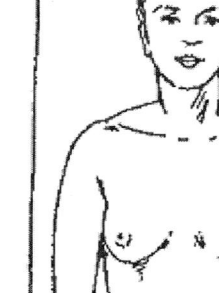

1. Stand before a mirror. Inspect both breasts for anything unusual, such as any discharge from the nipples or puckering, dimpling, or scaling of the skin. The next two steps are designed to emphasize any changes in the shape or contour of your breasts. As you do them, you should be able to feel your chest muscles tighten.

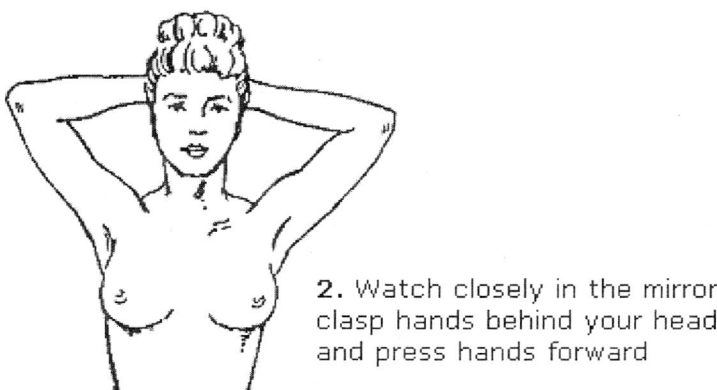

2. Watch closely in the mirror, clasp hands behind your head and press hands forward

3. Next, press hands firmly on hips and bow slightly towards the mirror as you pull your shoulders and elbows forward. Some women do the next part of the exam in the shower. Fingers glide over soapy skin, making it easy to concentrate on the texture underneath.

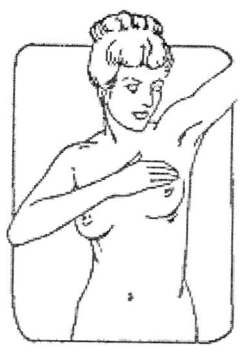

4. Raise your left arm. Use three or four fingers of your right hand to explore your left breast firmly, carefully, and thoroughly. Beginning at the outer edge, press the flat part of your fingers in small circles, moving the circles slowly around the breast. Gradually work toward the nipple. Be sure to cover the entire breast. Pay special attention to the area between the breast and the armpit itself. Feel for any unusual lump or mass under the skin.

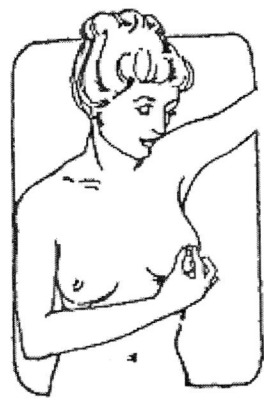

5. Gently squeeze the nipple and look for a discharge. Repeat the exam on your right breast.

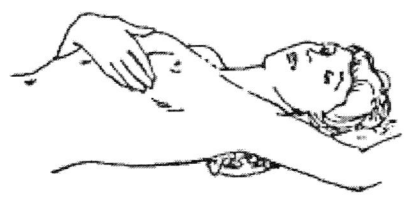

6. Repeat steps 4 and 5 lying down.
Lie flat on your back with your left arm over your head and a pillow or folded towel under your left shoulder. This position flattens the breast
and makes it easier to examine. Use the same circular motion described earlier.
Repeat on the right breast.

Medical Clearance

"Sweet April Showers, do Sweet May Flowers"

Thomas Tusser

From 1983 until the end of 1986, I was employed with WHO on short-term contracts because of medical restrictions. The contracts were for five months at a time, with breaks of more than 30 days. Then slowly but surely, and bit by bit, when my health behaved well, and I claimed no sick leaves during the short contracts, I was given longer short-term contracts in both the Public Information Office and the Division of Health and Biomedical Information.

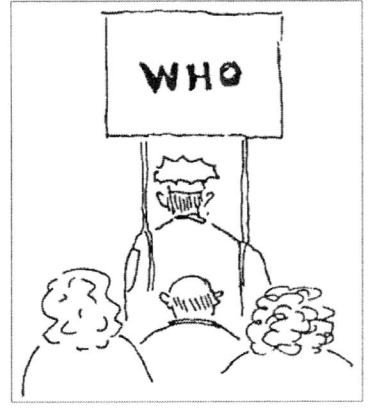

Then, unexpectedly, on a sunny winter day of the month of February 1987, I received in my in-tray together with the office mail, a sealed envelope addressed to me from the Personnel Officer of EMRO marked "PERSONAL AND STRICTLY CONFIDENTIAL". I grew pale, I could not open it, and I said to myself "Gosh! What did I write in EMROSA, that they are firing me for. I took a long breath, grabbed what was left of my courage and, opened the three-line letter.

"23 February 1987... Dear Mrs Allam, I am pleased to inform you that we have just received your medical clearance from headquarters. You may therefore apply for vacant long term posts, for which you qualify, as and when they are advertised .... With best wishes ... Yours sincerely, William R. Withee, Personnel Officer".

Only then did I feel that I was really back on my feet, and could consider myself an accredited member of the Organization, permitted to fly high the WHO flag. Although, I was never ever made to feel otherwise.

From 1987 until end 1990, I worked in a fixed-term post in the Office of External Coordination, where I gained more and more office experience and where I enjoyed editing "EMROSA" which had flourished by time, and had won fame throughout the regions.

I had never failed to periodically visit my doctor in Switzerland once a year. But one day in 1990, at his clinic in Geneva, the physician surprised me, "Mrs Allam" he said "now I can assure you that you will die of something else than breast cancer ... accordingly, I need not see you except once every ten years, if I am still alive ...".

My health, once condemned, had been cleared once by the World Health Organization in 1987, and now again, by the treating doctor who endorsed the judgment once more, adding to it some salt and pepper and some flavour too.

Geneva ... Again and Again

"The fates lead him who who will; him who won't they drag"

Old Persian saying

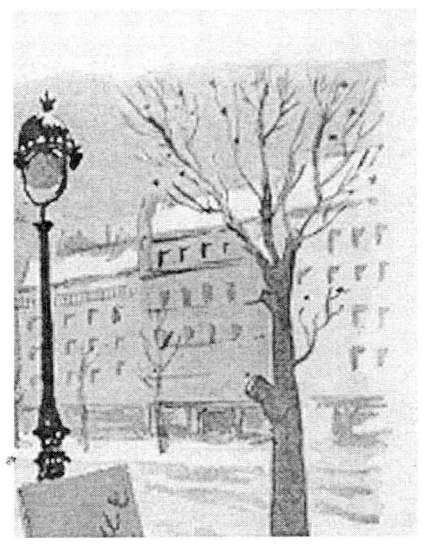

Call it coincidence or fate, illusion or fantasy, call it what you may, but definitely there exists a graspable attraction between the Swiss city and I. The big question is: "Does Geneva attract me or do I attract Geneva?"

When my doctor told me that he would see me once in ten years, I immediately thought that this was his problem. As for me, this place will always remain my recreation and "joie de vivre". Wondering, is it because deep inside me I felt that I was "re-created" in this cosmopolitan city or is it because it is where I was heavenly blessed? Frankly, I don't know and do not care to know.

To make a long story short, I left the physician's clinic and the first thing I did, I went right away to see the Personnel Officer at headquarters! I applied for a vacant post as and when available!

At that time, it was rare and unusual for general service staff members of WHO Regional Offices to apply for vacant posts in headquarters, Geneva. As 'pioneering' is a dominant trait of my personality, "I would never change," I thought. No way, I always look forward for a star that I would like to reach!

I went back home, resumed my normal life and my work in EMRO and forgot all about the daring application.

Strangely enough, two months later I received a letter from the Personnel department of headquarters inviting me for an interview for a vacant post in the Office of International Cooperation, WHO, Geneva!!

I praised and clapped my effervescent lucky stars. I took the plane to Geneva, went through a smooth interview, and by first January 1991, I started the duties of my post in Geneva, on the seventh floor - the lucky floor - behind a desk overlooking a panorama of paradise on earth.

By that time, my eldest son had obtained his B.Sc., in computer science and the younger one was working on his PhD., at McGill University, Canada. My husband could not "abandon ship"; I mean to say his work and profession. Nevertheless, he made frequent visits to Geneva and I to Alexandria. They say, absence makes the heart grow fonder.

I was successful in my job and well thought of by my superiors. I performed my duties whole-heartedly with patience and dedication and kept friendly and good relationships with all colleagues.

During my three-year stay in Geneva, I visited my doctor only once, when my eye caught a very small brown spot under my right arm. Although several of these are scattered elsewhere on my body, yet, the surgeon insisted to remove this particular one, which he did at his private clinic. It is no secret, at that time I thought the bells of danger were ringing again. I had a strange mix of surprise and fear. Thank God I have not heard those bells again.

Adding to my comfort was the circular issued by the WHO Geneva Staff Association commenting on the 1986 edition of my book,

> "cancer ... like all diseases, affects other people, never one's own family, and certainly not oneself. For we who deal with every kind of disease in terms of statistics every day, as our routine job, disease is

equated with incidence, mortality and morbidity, coverage of immunization, physicians per capita, any fact or figure which conveniently serves to depersonalize the whole business.

How many of us are prepared to stand up and say "I am depressive" (yes, WHO staff members also commit suicide); "I am an alcoholic"; "I have cancer"?

Luckily for our credibility, some do. And as our very own documents preach, self-awareness is the first step to a responsible attitude to disease, to facing up and giving doctors every chance to cure us. Our colleague, Nabila Allam, has been brave enough to make such a statement — and it is doubly difficult when it comes from a part of the world where lack of cancer awareness may deprive women of the chance of being cured if the disease is detected at an early stage.

Nabila has written a very personal moving account of her experience with breast cancer. It is a tribute to her personal courage and to the medical profession. Her aim is to demystify cancer, especially in those countries where the taboo of cancer prevents women from seeking treatment that is available to them, which could avoid wholly unnecessary personal tragedies ...

signed Mary Harper, Chairman, Staff Association, WHO Geneva

All the above and much more, helped my well-being, charged my batteries and kept me going strong.

Nostalgia

"In the middle of the journey of our life, I came to myself within a dark wood where the straight way was lost"

Dante Alighieri from the Divine Comedy

After three rewarding years of working in Geneva and after getting at the core of many international events, and mixing with an appealing cosmopolitan community, the nostalgia of returning home and the idea of living again among my family and amidst my friends overwhelmed me and began hunting me. The drums of nostalgia begun knocking hard, they attacked me on the hour, and gave way to many sleepless nights. I was asphyxiated. Healthy I was, but home sick I became. The symptoms started at the beginning of 1993.

The complexity of human nature is indeed incomprehensible. I felt I could not endure five more years until full retirement age.

In spite of the unbeatable Swiss coffee, and the unique entrecôte of "Café de Paris", in spite of the relatively high salary, and the promising stronger pension, my pencil started making calculations for the possibility of an early retirement at the end of the year.

Weighing and evaluating the positive and negative consequences in taking such a step, a decision had to be taken, a very difficult one indeed. I consulted with an Egyptian colleague of mine working under the same circumstances in Geneva, on whether if I put in my resignation and took early retirement people back home would call me a "silly girl". Astonished at the decision, unhesitant she said "Nabila ... it is you yourself who will look at the mirror and say, "What a stupid girl!". So, between "yes and no" and between "stupid girl" and "clever girl" the decision stayed in the balance for quite some time. Until one day the balance was adjusted.

"13 July 1993. ... Dear Mrs Allam ... Thank you for your memorandum dated 28 June 1993 from which I was sorry to learn that you wish to take early retirement and you will leave the Organization on 31 December 1993.

Your resignation is accepted with much regret ... The administrative services of Personnel will be glad to answer any questions you may have concerning formalities related to the termination of your appointment or to assist you in any other way. I should like to thank you for your contribution to the work of the Organization and to wish you well in the future ...

sgd. D. Pontz, Personnel Officer."

From the beginning of December, I felt I could not make it through to the end of the month! Drops in my blood pressure, irregular heart beats and unbearable headaches started haunting me. The WHO staff physician, with the "Staff Rules" in one hand, and the human "Psycho meter" in the other prescribed a highly effective medicine: a placebo. She exceptionally authorized me to leave the Organization on 15 December 1993.

The Healthier Side of Life

"Endings are beginnings in disguise"

Mexican proverb

January One, 1994,

I was back home amidst my family and among my friends. I have never ever regretted the decision or the step taken ... I am happy here.

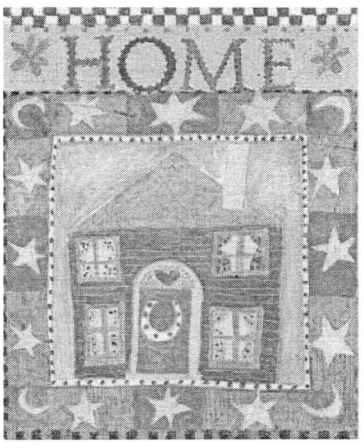

January One, 2003,

Over twenty years have so far elapsed since the operation; and I feel that these years have been the nicest, the best and the richest years of my life. I felt the touch of death ... now I sense the taste of life.

A lot can happen in twenty years. My eldest son joined EMRO nearly nine years ago; the younger one gave me a daughter-in-law and two lovely grandsons, Aly and Kamel, too.

Wednesday of every week, ten to fifteen EMRO retired staff members make a point of meeting over a cup of coffee at the Alexandria Sporting Club. We reminisce over our dear old days ... and WHO is always our favourite topic!

Let not the many events revealed in this book make me forget to assert how much I learned and how much I enjoyed working with WHO, both in EMRO and headquarters. I have always had a good salary, collaborative colleagues and supportive supervisors who helped me lead a more satisfactory and useful life.

Now that the past is far behind, I feel that I have reached my goals and captured my ideals.

I have reached and exceeded full retirement age, yet, I look younger than I should and I am still going strong. I have not so far suffered from any serious disease or illness, but if on the way, I run across a minor malaise, I make a point of seeing a physician at once, to avoid complex treatments, if any. May God forbid.

The Story has Ended

"... Much more could be done about cancer problems than most people believe. There is the knowledge to prevent a third of all existing cancers, to cure a third, if the cases are detected early enough, and to make sure that virtually all the incurable cases are spared pain..."*

---

* *Cancer Kit, Cancer Control Programme, World Health Organization, Geneva*